I0135263

Organic Perfumes

The Complete Guide To Making Simple
And Easy Homemade Organic Perfume

*(All Natural Organic Perfumes Recipes For
Beautiful Scent And Sweet Fragrances)*

Earl Johnson

Published By **Chris David**

Earl Johnson

All Rights Reserved

Organic Perfumes: The Complete Guide To Making Simple And Easy Homemade Organic Perfume (All Natural Organic Perfumes Recipes For Beautiful Scent And Sweet Fragrances)

ISBN   978-1-77485-509-6

No part of this guidebook shall be reproduced in any form without permission in writing from the publisher except in the case of brief quotations embodied in critical articles or reviews.

Legal & Disclaimer

The information contained in this ebook is not designed to replace or take the place of any form of medicine or professional medical advice. The information in this ebook has been provided for educational & entertainment purposes only.

The information contained in this book has been compiled from sources deemed reliable, and it is accurate to the best of the Author's knowledge; however, the Author cannot guarantee its accuracy and validity and cannot be held liable for any errors or omissions. Changes are periodically made to this book. You must consult your doctor or get professional medical advice before using any of the suggested remedies, techniques, or information in this book.

Upon using the information contained in this book, you agree to hold harmless the Author from and against any damages, costs, and expenses, including any legal fees potentially resulting from the application of any of the information provided by this guide. This disclaimer applies to any damages or injury caused by the use and application, whether directly or indirectly, of any advice or information presented, whether for breach of contract, tort, negligence, personal injury, criminal intent, or under any other cause of action.

You agree to accept all risks of using the information presented inside this book. You need to consult a professional medical practitioner in order to ensure you are both able and healthy enough to participate in this program.

Table of Contents

Introduction

This book provides the most effective ways and techniques to comprehend the theories and concepts behind the fascinating world of perfume production.

If you are willing to thoroughly read the book and then apply the knowledge contained in it this book, it will assist you in understanding the fundamentals of creating perfume using organic substances.

Making yourself a perfume can be an essential technique. Consumers who are conscious of their environment and budget will gain from learning how to create organic fragrances. The creative minds will love discovering this new form of art by mixing and matching essential oils to make something distinctive. When you are able to master this art you're no longer required to limit your choices of scents to the products of cosmetic firms.

The advantages of making your own organic fragrance are many! It's no as a surprise to learn that the commercial fragrances can be laced with the average of 29 harmful chemicals. When used for extended durations commercial perfumes can trigger serious health issues. Making your own natural perfumes will aid in protecting you and your family members from these risks. You can prevent the harmful adverse effect of harmful chemicals by learning to create your own fragrance.

An experienced perfumer invests the time and effort required to master the ability to blend scents that are irresistibly delicious. This book will teach you the basics of mixing essential oils as well as the steps involved in creating your own scent. After you have read these pages then you are able to begin searching for ingredients to create an aroma that is unique to yours.

Thank you for purchasing the book. I hope that you will enjoy it!

Chapter 1: The World Of Scents

Scents aren't visible, however they play a crucial role within our daily lives. They are essential to our existence and is connected to fundamental human interactions such as eating and mating. It is possible to use the senses of smell appreciate expensive perfumes or to know what is suitable to consume. It is able to tell whether something is burning or smells dirty. It doesn't matter if you know that or not, human beings can recognize the smell of 10,000 different things. Your nose could be telling you more than you think.

The effect of smell is undervalued. Certain scents can make an enormous impact on relaxation, sleep and improvement of mood. You can dramatically improve you mood as well as create positive mood if you're aware of how various scents perform.

Our ancestors discovered the wonders of smells when they discovered the possibilities with the help of fire. Through throwing leaves, herbs and twigs as well as other plant material into flames they were able to create diverse smells which were both good and bad. The creation of colognes and perfumes has an interesting background. Our ancestors from the past also used perfumes for funerals and religious rituals to connect with gods and deceased.

Perfumery, also known as the art of creating fragrances, is believed to begin in Egypt. While perfumes played a significant part in the various rituals but they also played a role to heal and for the decoration of daily life. They became more popular when the methods of perfumery were handed down into the Greeks. People began to add fragrances in their daily routines for hygiene.

Through the 18th and 19th centuries the perfumery industry became more sophisticated and more modern. The development of chemistry as well as other techniques of science led to an evolution in the way perfumes were created. This made it possible for greater access to fragrances. Today, fragrance is seen as an accessory to fashion, and is commonly used to enhance the appearance that the person wearing it.

Statistics indicate that both males and females alike have an interest in buying perfumes. Around 80 percent of people purchase scents at least once in a year! It's fascinating that perfumes of today continue to draw customers.

The perfume industry is making money. It's relatively inexpensive to create a scent however, the cost of perfumes are expensive. One reason for the huge success of the perfume business is its sense of scent's ability. The scent of perfume can trigger memories and emotions. A smelt of crayons could make you think of fond memories of your childhood. The scent of baking bread could make you feel fuller than you actually are. In a way, the smell is a great way to transport yourself to another place and time.

Scent also reveals something about the person wearing it. It can be a significant factor in the person's appearance. A scent that is pleasant makes a great impression. When you're out for your first date or at an interview for your final job it's important to select the scent that's suitable for you.

Many of us have our own personal scents. You may also be at risk of spraying yourself in scents of your favourite perfume before leaving the house. Unfortunately, perfumes that are manufactured for commercial use pose a serious health risk. There are many issues that arise from the usage of fragrances. Apart from the cost many perfumes are constructed of harmful substances. In the long term the use of perfumes can pose negative health hazards for the person who wears it, to those around him or her as well as to the surrounding environment.

The Risks of Perfume Use

Your desire for smelling nice could be doing much more damage than you imagine. However all of the "mildest" fragrances can trigger allergic reactions to the skin and allergies that could cause serious health issues in the end. Watery eyes and sneezing are the most commonly reported adverse reaction to fragrance. Dermatitis and skin conditions are also fairly frequent. In the most severe cases, allergies to perfume can be a cause of depression too.

General irritation, which is characterized by an inflamed and red skin could be the result of the irritants in perfumes with harsh chemicals. People with sensitive skin could develop eczema, or chronic skin disorders. Strangely enough, such cases are not uncommon. Around one-tenth of people are thought to be allergic to fragrance chemicals.

Researchers have even suggested that perfumes can cause hormonal disruption. The estrogen and parabens are believed to be in up to 75 percent of fragrances available on the market in the present. While estrogen is a natural component in the body however exposure to an abnormally large amount can lead to the development of breast cancer. Parabens pose a similar risk. They are associated with illnesses in various organs like kidneys, the liver and lungs.

The most surprising part is the simple fact that one doesn't have to put on the scent to be able to harm your body. Inhaling it can be enough to cause harm. The chemicals found in commercial perfumes can be harmful for mothers who are breastfeeding as they can pass onto babies. You could be contributing to your children's skin or allergy issues without knowing it!

Additionally the store-bought fragrances are recognized to harm the environment, too. Synthetic fragrances are laced with harmful chemicals that evaporate into the air with each spray. Fish, in particular could ingest the harmful chemicals and put them at risk as well. In addition, if excessive amounts of these chemicals end up in our tap water there could be severe side effects that could lead to health issues.

If you could choose to use perfumes which are made of natural substances instead of toxic chemicals it's easy to decide which are suitable for use, isn't it?

It's actually not that easy.

Scents are classified as trade secrets. So, perfume manufacturers do not have to disclose the chemicals they employed in the creation of scents. The only way is to determine which perfumes have the most dangerous chemicals. It is difficult to make an informed choice when information isn't readily accessible.

What should you do? Should you quit using perfumes?

Not at all! It is all you need to do is learn to make your own natural fragrances.

Make Your Own Fragrance

There are many advantages to creating your personal perfume. Because you control the ingredients that you are using it is possible to ensure that pesticides, chemicals or other harmful substances will not be added to your formula. Apart from reducing the risks of skin irritation and allergies as well as avoiding nausea, migraines and irritation to the lungs due to commercially-available perfumes. You'll surely gain from mastering this technique.

The organic perfumes made of natural ingredients and are suitable for all. Children too have the "go" signal make use of organic perfumes since they do not contain chemicals that are absorbed by the skin and later in the bloodstream.

In addition to health benefits organic perfumes are beneficial for your body since they provide both emotional and physical advantages. Since organic fragrances are generally made of essential oils you will be able to enjoy the relaxing, healing and uplifting properties that come from organic ingredients. It is possible to boost your mood by spraying your personal blend of perfume.

In addition, using organic fragrances can allow you to create a unique scent. Organic perfumes don't completely cover the natural scent of the wearer like synthetic perfumes can. Organic perfumes react with your body, creating a unique scent that isn't artificial or overpowering.

By grasping the fundamentals of essential oils as well as the fundamentals of perfumery, you'll be able to quickly create a fragrance from your own home at the convenience of your home. You don't require the expertise of a specialist or any specific equipment. If you have a basic understanding of essential oils, and a keen sense of smell to know what smells good, you can make your own organic scent.

Chapter 2: Essentials Of Essential Oils

Mixing essential oils to create a pleasant fragrance is a blend of science and art. Although creating your own perfume might appear complex at first, don't fool yourself. It's actually quite simple. All you require is the essential oils, along with several other essential perfumery ingredients and you'll be well on your way. You can also create your personal organic perfume in just only 24 hours or less.

Making your own scent is a great exercise to stimulate your senses. Making a variety of essential oils can allow you to discover scents that awaken your sexuality. It's a fun pastime which will allow you to develop your creativity. It will help you save dollars, and you could even make perfumes for loved ones to give as gifts. Your personal fragrance is guaranteed to be personalised and completely individual. You can't find anything similar to it in any cosmetic store or on the internet.

Before you know how to make perfume, you must know the fundamentals about essential oils. Since the beginning of time essential oils were used to enhance the beauty of your skin. Essential oils are extremely concentrated and extremely fragrant. They are made up of around a hundred varieties of chemicals that come that come from plants. The diversity of the natural chemicals within essential oils makes them so valuable.

Essential oils are extremely complex. They can aid to find a sense balance in a manner that none of the synthetic perfumes can. Essential oils smell pleasant and natural and usually stimulate the brain's center of activity for emotional and mental memory. If you choose the appropriate essential oils, you will feel more calm or you can boost your mood. This is more valuable than anything synthetic perfume can provide you with.

To truly experience the relaxing and healing properties of essential oils make sure you purchase the purest quality of essential oil you can lay the chance to get. If you can, you should try to get 100% natural essential oils. These are ones that have no additives or removed when extracting them. The more pure the oils are and the more pure the scents will be. They may be more expensive however they'll make you feel and smell better.

Essential oils may be distinguished by their smell. Certain scents are floral (like Jasmine and lavender) while others are fruity (like lemon, citrus and lime) as well as more woody (like the pine or cedar). Although there aren't any strict guidelines to mixing essential oils, certain scents that belong in the same group typically work well together.

The best part is that there aren't any strict and unambiguous rules that must be adhered to when the mixing of essential oils. Anyone who is looking to make perfumes can mix and mix scents until they discover a scent that fits their preferences and personality.

Chemical Chemistry and Essential Oils Chemistry of Essential Oils

Fragrances that are applied to your body right now won't smell exactly the same as they do three hours later. This is the case with both commercially produced perfumes as well as organic fragrances. This is why having a basic understanding of chemistry will help in understanding how perfumery works. Certain scents are more likely to evaporate than others. As a scent disappear, the scent that remains shifts. It is essential to consider what scents you wish to fade faster and what scents you would like to stay for a longer time.

Perfumes comprise three layers comprising base notes middle notes, top notes. They are classified by length of time the fragrance is expected to last. The top notes can take anywhere from 1 to 2 hours to go away. Middle notes can take up to four up to eight hours for them to disappear and bases notes will be the ones that last. Some of the most robust base notes will last for many days!

Understanding Perfume Notes

Top notes

First impressions are the most lasting, therefore it is essential to ensure that you select your top notes carefully. The top notes are the initial explosion of scent that the perfume emits. You'll notice the top notes from the moment the scent is absorbed by your skin. Essential oils of the floral and citrus families are typically employed to create top-notes.

Here are a few of the most popular choices for the top notes:

Lavender - Lavender flowers are popular for their relaxing effect. You can add lavender essential oil with your perfume if you wish to feel calm and relaxed when you spray your scent. It's also beneficial to apply lavender as it is an acknowledged enhancer. It can help make other essential oils smell more appealing. In reality, lavender is an amazing treat for your sense of smell.

Mandarin or Orange-Sweet. These essentials from the citrus family are sure to add a refreshing scent to your perfume! They are very sultry and possess both familiarity and depth. They're best paired with powerful mid notes and base notes. Jasmine and Vetiver are great for the top note of citrus.

CarnationCarnation Carnation is a luxurious and lavish scent. If you wear this fragrance, you'll be awed. Carnation flowers usually smell more delicate and more delicate than carnation essential oils. While this scent may be slightly more expensive than other scents, you are certain to get a pleasant experience!

Cinnamon- The smell of cinnamon is sweet and sweet. It is considered to be extremely valuable since it has been proven to combat depression and exhaustion. It's extremely energizing and helps to energize people who feel weak.

Peppermintis refreshing and sharp fragrance of menthol. It is often linked with increased alertness in the mind and concentration. The minty scent is well-known to ease the skin and reduce redness and irritation. Peppermint is a great choice for people who want to feel youthful refreshed, fresh and rejuvenated.

Mid Notes

Mid notes are regarded as the essence of fragrance. They help balance the scent and also assist in getting rid of unpleasant smells or blends. Some perfumers view the mid notes to be the essence of the fragrance. This is what gives the perfume its distinctive smell. Pick stronger scents that create a lasting impression as they are absorbed into the skin.

Here are some great mid notes alternatives:

Roserose Rose is perhaps one of the most valuable essential oils you can find. It is recognized by its distinctive fragrance that is not too subtle nor too strong. It's sensual, and is an extremely well-known as an aphrodisiac. Be cautious if the cost for the oil that you buy isn't enough. Essential rose oil can be a little more expensive than other brands and has an excellent reason!

Jasminejasmine Jasmine is a popular option for mid-tones. It is a little stronger than the majority of essential oils that are formal, however it has a distinct relaxing impact that gives it a strong and intense scent. It has an exotic ambiance. Much like the rose, it's also sensual, and an as aphrodisiac. It's a good match for the fruity notes of mango or citrus.

Neroli- Neroli is not as well-known as the other oils that are essential, however this scent is extremely beneficial because it's believed for its ability to combat depression. It is the result of the blossom of the tree of orange, and so it is a refreshing citrus smell. It's very refreshing, however it gives off the sensation of a delicate and sophisticated sensation.

Chamomileis a Chamomile is a well-known for its fruity, sweet scent. It can be calming when you are annoyed or frustrated. A small amount of chamomile essential oil is needed to create a powerful aroma.

Geranium- Geranium has become a extremely popular essential oil. It helps maintain the equilibrium between the mind and emotions. It can have a uplifting effect which is a huge help in tackling emotional stress and anxiety. The scent has been proven to assist women with depression and premenstrual syndrome.

Base notes

The fundamental scent that you choose for your scent is primary thing you need to choose when you're thinking about the essential oils you want to mix. It is the scent which will last for the longest time. In addition regardless of whether it's simply the "background" for the middle note and the top one, it's typically very strong, and it's supposed to intensify the scents of the other notes, particularly the middle note. A strong base note is essential to recognizing any perfume.

There are only a handful of fragrances that perfumers usually change when it comes back to the basic note, as there are only a handful of scents that are strong enough to last for a lengthy period of.

Here are a few of the most well-known most popular:

Patchouliis a popular scent. Patchouli is a very well-known essential oil and its scent is utilized in many different household products. It's a great base note due to its an intense, strong scent that lasts for a long period of time. In its own form the smell of patchouli isn't particularly extraordinary. When combined with other oils, it can be very pleasant in smell. If you feel you think patchouli is too intense for you, consider trying the vetiver alternative.

Vanilla- The familiar scent is very soothing scent that is very soothing. It's soft and warm and will leave the wearer with a scent and feel sexually attractive. Vanilla has a soothing and soothing impact. It's surprising, but it's a good match with fruity and floral essential oils.

Sandalwood- Unlike bases, sandalwood isn't extremely powerful. It is nevertheless guaranteed to be extremely sexually attractive and sexually sexy. It makes an impression since it can feel extremely sensual and luxurious. It also can be mixed well with other essential oils from the fruity and floral families.

Vetiver-Vetriver oil is a well-known essential oil that is known for its ability to rejuvenate the body in a complete way. It is a relaxing oil that is helpful in the elimination of anger, stress or other hostile emotions. Vetiver is renowned for its healing and rejuvenating effects. If you're looking to relieve tension, then this could be the best option for you.

Ylang-ylang: The calming floral scent of ylang ylang is delicious and exotic. It's known to reduce tension and fatigue. The strong scent is wonderful by itself, however it's best mixed with lighter scents like Bergamot.

Chapter 3: How To Make Your Own Perfume

Apart from essential oils, you'll also require other products that will be required to create your own scent that is organic. These ingredients are also helpful in other projects to do it yourself So don't be concerned about the initial expense. Additionally, it's highly likely that the cost of these components would be more expensive than what we typically spend on perfumes. Even if you indulge a little it won't cost you the amount.

In addition to essential oils, here are other essential items you need to need to begin your organic perfume creation.

Pure grain alcohol Vodka is the most effective Emulsifier for organic perfumes. 100 proof is ideal however any type of vodka can be used. If you're using a vodka that is lower in percentage, you should shake it before you use it. Because you won't be drinking it It's fine to purchase cheap brands.

GlycerinThere is no consensus among experts that glycerin is a must-have ingredient for the production of organic perfumes, however for those who are just beginning this ingredient is extremely beneficial. Glycerin can help the mix retain its scent. If you're just beginning your journey it is possible to incorporate this into your mix to ensure that the fragrance last. Once you've become proficient at mixing oils with essentials you could find yourself creating more of a base can give the similar result. Glycerin can be easily found in pharmacies.

Distilled or spring water It is essential to make use of spring or distillated water to eliminate any contamination that might impact your mixture. Tap water typically contains lead and minerals, which could impact the other components in your mix. It typically gives the body scent and, if utilized in the correct quantity, it's unlikely to alter the fragrance of the mix.

Bottling supplies- You require bottling materials to keep your scent over a long duration of. It is vital to ensure that all the materials you uses is clean to prevent impurities from entering your mix. A sterilized bottle, coffee filter and a sprayer will assist you in packaging your scent.

How to Make your own perfume

After you've prepared your ingredients, you're ready to begin making your personal perfume.

1. Mix your essential oils

When you're just beginning, you're at liberty to experiment with the combinations and proportions that are appealing to you. That's how to find the best combinations. Enjoy looking for scents that appeal to you. Here are some recommended proportions to mix your notes of perfume.

Six to eight drops of base note

10-15 drops in middle notes.

9.12 drops of high notes

Naturally, you are able to experiment with these ratios until you find an aroma that is distinctive. If you'd like you to, you can make use of any middle note or top note. Any combination you like is fine. Do not be shackled by rules, and revel in the freedom of mixing various scents.

2. Mix your essential oil in with the other ingredients

Then, mix your essential oils with other ingredients that are needed to create your fragrance. The ratios typically range from 15-30 per cent essential oils. 70-80 percent vodka, and five percent of distillated water. It is however not a set formula. Many people like to play with the proportions and mix the ingredients however they feel is appropriate.

You can mix the essential oil along with the vodka in the beginning and let it rest for about 12 hours. The length of time that you keep your scent is contingent on the amount of duration you've got. It is possible to age it for up to 6 days if you prefer an ominous fragrance. It is important that during the process of aging it is stored in a dry, cool area.

After the process of aging After the aging process, determine what amount of water that will be required based on the strength of the fragrance. If you're just beginning adding Glycerin to keep the scent longer. However, as you get better at mixing oils, you'll eventually discover the ideal blend which will enable you to boost the strength of your scent simply by using essential oils.

3. You can play around with the recipe

If you're happy with the smell of your perfume after your first go, be sure to note down the formula so that you will be able to recreate the scent. If you're not satisfied with the scent, you may experiment until you find something that is truly satisfying to your sense of scent.

In reality there are likely to be thousands of combinations can be easily accessed on the internet. If you're getting bored by the experiments you're trying you can "cheat" to a degree. Find a recipe that is interesting. Record the recipes you love. It's the only way to be able replicate the aromas you truly enjoy.

4. Eliminate the scent

All kinds of dirt or impurities are sure to impact the scent and the shelf life the perfume. You must ensure that you eliminate undesirable foreign substances prior to moving your perfume into its appropriate bottles. Utilize a simple cheesecloth or coffee filter to clean and filter your perfume.

5. Transfer to bottles

Now you're accomplished! Simply transfer the fragrance into bottles and then cover it by covering it with a spray cap. To create a greater impact it is possible to create names for your fragrance. This is a great idea for presents for Christmas to your beloved family members and friends.

Making a solid Perfume

In the present day many perfumes are available in liquid form, however there was an era that solid perfumes were in the fashion. If you're looking to make something that has a distinct and authentic feel. You could make an actual perfume instead.

The process of essential oils will be generally the similar, but you will need to add two essential ingredients that alter the scent such as beeswax and carrier oil. For perfumes that are solid there is no need to make use of alcohol and aren't required to let your blend sit for a long period of time.

Below are some steps to making a perfume for sale:

Mix the beeswax with the carrier oil.

The most common rule is mixing equal amounts of carrier oil and beeswax. If you plan to make use of 2 tablespoons beeswax you need to make use of 2 tablespoons of the carrier oil, too. The most popular carrier oils include the olive oil of almonds Jojoba oil, as well as grape seed oil.

In the future, if you find that the mix is too thick, increase the amount of carriers oil till you have the consistency you'd like.

Make Essential Oils

Make the essential oils the same manner as described in the previous paragraph. Mix both the middle and top notes, and base notes the same way.

It is also possible to make containers to store your soaps. In lieu of bottles keep your scent in tiny tin containers. If you intend to give them away as presents, you can opt for elaborate vintage locks or containers for a an authentic appearance.

Melt the Beeswax

After you've prepared everything and are ready to begin melt the mixture of beeswax by using the double-broiler. If you don't own a double-broiler simply place the beeswax blend in a container that is heat-safe. Put it in a pot with boiling liquid to soften the wax. The beeswax melts at a low temperature , and continue stirring until the mixture melts.

It is possible to mix in the essential oil after all of the beeswax is completely melted. Continue to stir to ensure that the oils essential are evenly distributed.

Pour the mixture in the containers while they're still warm. When they have solidified, warm the mixture again.

Chapter 4: Tips On Perfumery And

Techniques

Like any other skill it takes patience and perseverance for mastering the craft and the process behind the art of perfume making. It's unlikely that you'll become awestruck by the first fragrance you make. There's the possibility that you'll need to make several batches before you discover the perfect scent that pleases your senses.

In the hope of making the initial few attempts easier to you, below are a few suggestions to help you when you begin.

Don't Let Yourself Be Disillusioned

Remember that you're making natural perfumes made of natural substances. It is far too high to assume that it will smell exactly similar to the synthetic perfume you wore every day. Because your perfume is made of pure ingredients, the scent won't produce the same effects like the perfumes you purchase on the market.

Set your expectations in a reasonable manner. Try not to replicate your preferred synthetic perfume. Since you're working with natural substances, it might not be feasible to keep the scent for a long time. The scent will also be somewhat different to those which are available. Don't get discouraged! Sooner or later, you'll discover your groove and create scents that appeal to your sense of scent.

It is also advisable to make small quantities when you are just beginning your journey. It could be a bit painful to create many bottles of a certain scent only to find out that you're not pleased with the scent. Try it out and then create a huge batch after you've perfected the recipe.

Your sense of smell will Change

Once you are familiar with working with and using natural fragrances You will notice that your sense of smell begins to shift dramatically. You'll be more sensitive to scents and you'll not be a fan of the fake scent that is emitted by synthetic fragrances.

You'll gain an understanding of the process of creating perfume as you learn the importance of essential oils. Find out which smells you love. Define the elements of the scents that interest you. Discover the blends you really like. Discover the different smells as well as their categories. This will help you be more confident when you create your own mixtures.

It is also good to know what essential oils "smell alike" so that you know what alternatives you can use in case your first choice is not available. If you know what other scents belong to the same family, you'll find it easier to find a replacement for whatever ingredient is missing. Small Doses do not Equate to a Small Impact

If you like a particular scent, resist the urge to throw large doses of the essential oil into your perfume. Remember that you don't need a huge amount to create impact. In fact, if you put in too much, it might be too overpowering. With some of the stronger oils, even a small amount can create a strong scent.

Make Your Perfumes More Attractive

There are a variety of ways to make your perfume much more attractive. If you want to add an interesting color to your perfumes, you can add all-natural vegetable dye to your mixture. It won't affect the scent of your perfume, but it will make it more visually appealing.

You can also add petals to make your perfume look more interesting. Though petals will only glve a minimal contribution to the scent, it will give your perfume a more exotic overall appearance.

Bottle your perfume nicely. For long-term storage, a dark-colored bottle is your best option. Make sure that direct sunlight does not fall on our perfume. Some even like to refrigerate their perfumes in order to make it last longer.

Know How to Wear Your Perfumes

Knowing how to wear your scents means knowing how much to spray and where to spray. Spray too much and the scent will be too overpowering. Spray too little and you might not appreciate your scent. The right amount sprayed on the right area will enhance the scent of your perfume.

Since you are using an organic perfume, you might have to spray the perfume more often because the scent of organic perfume generally doesn't last as long as the scent of synthetic perfume. You can try spraying on key points of the body to see if spraying on these areas will make the scent last longer. The known key points are the wrists, behind your ears and behind the knees. Since you are using organic scents, you don't have to worry about the perfume touching your skin. Those who really want their scents to last longer can opt to spray on their hair and clothes instead.

Chapter 5: Toxic Free Divine Smelling

Perfumes

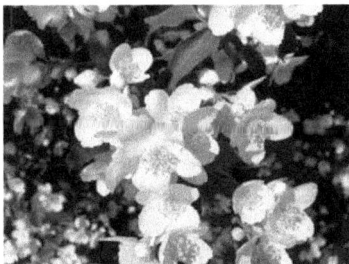

There are a few recipes that will help you to make Toxic Free Divine Smelling Perfumes at your own home. These recipes are easy to follow for everyone:

Recipe 01: Jasmine Perfume

- Jojoba Oil: 2 tablespoons

- Distilled water: 1 tablespoon

- Jasmine: 30 drops

- Vanilla: 5 drops

- Lavender: 5 drops

Directions:

Mix all essential oils in one glass bottle and keep this bottle aside for almost two days. Mix in distilled water and shake them well. Leave this blend for nearly four weeks in one dark and cool spot. In the case of any sediment, you can strain this mixture through a cheese cloth. Pour it in a spray bottle and enjoy.

Recipe 02: Natural Perfume

- Jojoba Oil: 1 oz

- Distilled water: 1 oz

- Jasmine oil: 5 drops

- Lemon oil: 3 drops

- Orange oil: 3 drops

- Sandalwood oil: 3 drops

Directions:

Combine all ingredients in one small container and mix them well by tipping the bottle up and down. You can apply it on the neck, behind your ear or wrist. It will keep you fresh and fragrant for almost 2 to 3 hours.

Recipe 03: Rose Petal Perfume

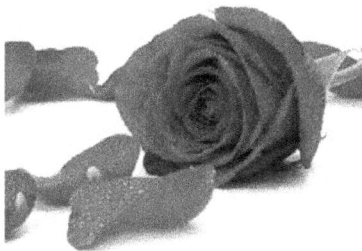

You will need almost 30 – 35 petals of rose with strong fragrance.

Put these petals in one cup and fill this cup with water to soak all petals. Strain this water, but secure these rose petals. Put them in pastel-and-mortar and mash these petals to grind them.

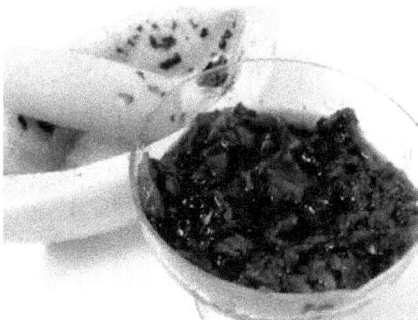

Put these grind petals in strained water and once again strain moisture from petals. Continue this procedure until the water becomes brownish-pinkish-orangish color. Now take out all rose petals and enjoy this rose water. You can put it in a spray bottle.

Recipe 04: Organic Flower Perfume

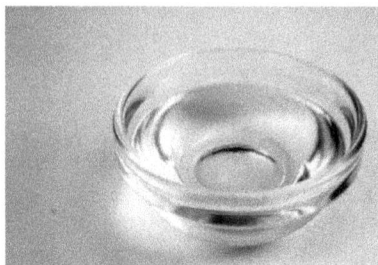

- Chopped flowers: 1 1/2 cups
- Glass bowl with lid

- Cheesecloth

- Small saucepan

- Distilled water: 2 cups

- Sterilize a glass bottle with airtight cap

Directions:

You can take the petals of your favorite flower and wash them to remove sediment and dirt with water.

You have to soak flowers and put cheesecloth in the bowl with edges. The cheesecloth should overlap the bowl. You can put flowers in the cheesecloth-lined bowl and carefully pour water on petals to cover these flowers. Cover this bowl with one lid and place this bowl aside for one night.

In the next day, remove the lid of the bowl and slowly join the four corners of the cheesecloth and lift the pouch of flowers from this water bowl. Squeeze this pouch on the saucepan and extract scented water. Simmer this water on low heat until only one teaspoon liquid left.

Put this perfume in the bottle and secure its cap. This fragrance can be used for one month. You should secure it in a dark and cold place.

Recipe 05: Lavender Scent

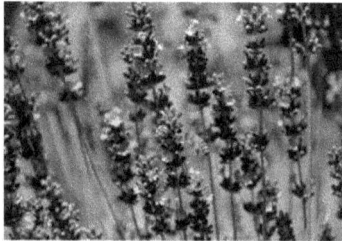

- Distilled Water
- Plastic Bottle

- 3 Lavender flower and 1 red rose

- Eye dropper

Directions:

Remove buds and petals from rose and lavender flowers. Wash all flower petals to remove mud. Add petals in the cooking pan in the boiling water and reduce heat to let it simmer. After 15 minutes, pour this water along with buds and petals in a jug to cool down.

Now use cheesecloth to strain scented water, and throw petals and buds. The water will be turned pink in color and the petals should be white. You can use an eye dropper or pipette to transfer this perfume to a perfume atomizer. The perfume is ready to use.

Recipe 06: Fragrance of Rose and Clove

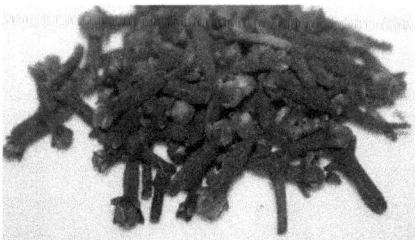

- Jojoba oil: 1/4 cup

- Clove oil: 2 to 3 drops

- Rose oil: 1 teaspoon

- Dark glass bottle

Directions:

Take one dark bottle to because it is good to secure your perfume. Blend all ingredients (except clove) and mix them well. You can pour this mixture at least 12 hours. Clove can overpower other ingredients; therefore, you can add it in the last and pour one drop at one time. Select a cool and dry area to store it. You can dab it on pulse points to enjoy the long-lasting fragrance. You can increase the amount of rose oil to make the scent strong.

Recipe 07: Orange and Mint Cologne

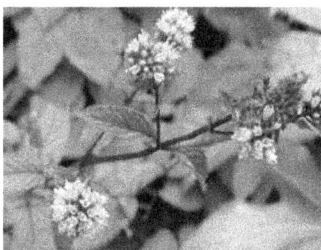

- Orange peel (remove white pith): 1 orange

- Mint leaves: a handful

- Sweet citrus EO (essential oil): 5 drops

- Peppermint EO: 1 drop

- Vodka (optional)

Directions:

Take a clean mason jar and combine mint and orange peel in one Mason jar. Pour vodka or distilled water in the jar and put the lid back. Shake this jar well and leave for almost 4 to 6 weeks. The cologne is ready, and now you can add sweet citrus and peppermint in one cup of cologne. You can pour this blend in one spray bottle for later use.

Chapter 6: Organic Perfumes With Flowers And Essential Oil

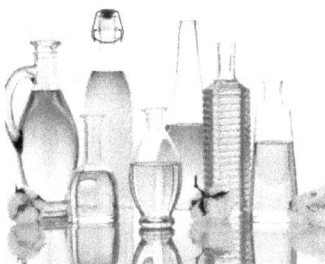

There are some essential oils that prove good to make organic perfumes. These perfumes are good for your skin.

Recipe 08: Romantic Perfume

- Cedarwood EO: 3 drops

- Bergamot EO: 15 drops

- Sandalwood: 3 drops

- 100 proof vodka (optional): 300ml

- 2 drops vanilla EO

Directions:

First add vodka (if using) in one jar and put all the ingredients and shake them well. It will be good to secure this mixture in a dark bottle and put this bottle in one dark and cool place for almost 7 days. You can rub it on your pulse points to enjoy the enduring fragrance.

Recipe 09: Sandalwood Perfume

- Water (distilled): 2 cups

- Perpetual essential oil: 5 drops

- 100 Proof vodka: 3 tablespoons

- Sandalwood EO: 10 drops

- Peony EO: 10 drops

Directions:

In the first step, add vodka (if using) in one jar and put all the ingredients and shake them well. It will be good to secure this mixture in a dark bottle and put this bottle in one dark and cold place for almost seven days. You can rub it on your pulse points to enjoy the enduring fragrance.

Recipe 10: Mesmerizing Blend

- Water (distilled): 2 cups

- Sandalwood EO: 5 drops

- Vodka or Grape fruit EO: 3 tablespoons

- Cassis EO: 10 drops

- Bergamot EO: 10 drops

Directions:

In the first step, add vodka (if using) in one jar and put all the ingredients and shake them well. It will be good to secure this mixture in a dark bottle and put this bottle in one dark and cold place for almost seven days. You can rub it on your pulse points to enjoy the enduring fragrance.

Recipe 11: Lilly Aromatic Oil

- Lilly flowers: 12

- Sweet almond EO: 20 drops

Directions:

Take a jar and put oil and lily flowers in this jar. Cover this jar and put aside for almost 24 hours. You can use a wooden spoon to press down flowers to release their fragrance. After 24 hours, you can use funnel to strain flowers. If you want strong scent, you can increase flowers and infusion time. Seal this jar to keep it away from sunlight. You can use this oil as massage or bath oil.

Recipe 12: Extract Rose Water at Home

- Fresh roses: 2 (1 cup petals)

- Distilled water: 2 cups

- Vodka (it is optional): 1 teaspoon

Directions:

You should have fresh roses and wash them properly to remove any insects and pesticides. Put these petals in the saucepan and soak in distilled water. It is time to add vodka and cover the pan with its lid and keep it on low heat. There is no need to let them boil or simmer because it can ruin the actual properties of rose. Wait for almost 20 minutes, until the water change its color. It is time to strain this liquid in a mason jar and close its lid. This jar can be stored in your refrigerator for almost seven days.

Recipe 13: Chamomile Bled

- Water (distilled): 2 cups

- Rose oil: 5 drops

- Valerian oil: 10 drops

- Chamomile oil: 10 drops

- Body glitter (as per need)

Directions:

In the first step, take one jar and put all the ingredients and shake them well. It will be good to secure this mixture in a dark bottle and put this bottle in one dark and cold place for almost seven days. You can rub it on your pulse points to enjoy the enduring fragrance.

Recipe 14: Rosemary Perfume

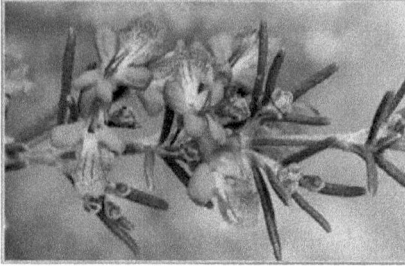

- Water (distilled): 2 cups

- Hypericum EO: 5 drops

- Rosemary EO: 10 drops

- Cypress EO: 10 drops

- Vodka (optional): 3 tablespoons

Directions:

In the first step, add vodka (if using) in one jar and put all the ingredients and shake them well. It will be good to secure this mixture in a dark bottle and put this bottle in one dark and cold place for almost

seven days. You can rub it on your pulse points to enjoy the enduring fragrance.

Recipe 15: Misty Perfume

- Ylang-ylang EO: 2 drops
- Passionflower EO: 3 drops
- Neroli EO: 3 drops
- Vodka (optional): 1/2 part (300ml)

Directions:

In the first step, add vodka (if using) in one jar and put all the ingredients and shake them well. It will be good to secure this mixture in a dark bottle and put this bottle in one dark and cold place for almost seven days. You can rub it on your pulse points to enjoy the enduring fragrance.

Recipe 16: Bergamot Perfume

- Water (distilled): 2 cups
- Sandalwood EO: 5 drops

- Vodka (optional): 3 tablespoons

- Cassis rose oil: 10 drops

- Bergamot EO: 10 drops

Direction:

In the first step, add vodka (if using) in one jar and put all the ingredients and shake them well. It will be good to secure this mixture in a dark bottle and put this bottle in one dark and cold place for almost seven days. You can rub it on your pulse points to enjoy the enduring fragrance.

Recipe 17: Good Night Perfume

- Musk EO (organic): 4 drops

- Sandalwood EO: 4 drops

- Jojoba oil: 2 teaspoons

- Frankincense EO: 3 drops

Directions:

In the first step, add vodka (if using) in one jar and put all the ingredients and shake them well. It will be good to secure this mixture in a dark bottle and put this bottle in one dark and cold place for almost seven days. You can rub it on your pulse points to enjoy the enduring fragrance.

Chapter 7: Solid Perfumes For Him And Her

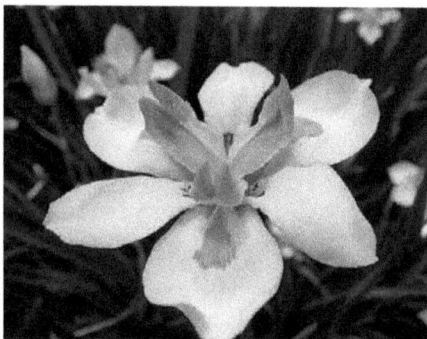

If you want solid perfumes, there are a few recipes to make your own solid perfumes. These solid blends will be great for everyone:

Recipe 18: Jasmine Fragrance

- Fresh Jasmine flowers: 1 medium bowl
- Moisturizing cream

Directions:

You can use any moisturizing cream as per your skin. Take a wide jar and cover it with a thick layer of cream (the pot should be wide enough to put your hand comfortably in this pot. Fill the jar with flowers and cover each corner of this jar with flowers. Secure the lid and keep it for almost one month. It is important to regularly change the jasmine flowers and throw old one in dustbin. After one month, you can check the jar and smell this cream. If the fragrance is strong, you can remove flowers and mix this cream with other cream for later use.

Recipe 19: Solid Perfume

- Grapefruit EO: 17 drops
- Ginger EO: 14 drops
- Beeswax pastilles: 1 tablespoon

- Vetiver essential oil: 10 drops

Directions:

Use microwave or double boiler to melt the beeswax. It is time to mix all essential oils in the beeswax. You have to pour this mixture in one jar or bottle. It is easy to pour solid perfume in a heart-shaped or round locket to keep it always with you.

Recipe 20: Almond Oil Solid Perfume

- Beeswax: 1 tablespoon
- Almond oil: 1 tablespoon
- Glass container: 1
- Straw: 1
- Pyrex bowl or glass jar for mixing: 1
- Saucepan: 1
- Orange EO: 6 drops
- Ylang-ylang EO: 4 drops
- Bergamot oil: 4 drops
- Rosewood EO: 3 drops
- Frankincense oil: 3 drops

- Jasmine oil: 2 drops

Directions:

Collect ingredients and supplies before starting you work. Measure out almond oil and wax in the glass jar. Put one inch water in a saucepan and place the bowl or jar containing wax in this water. Let this water boil to gradually melt wax.

Once the wax turn into liquid, you can remove it from heat. Mix in essential oils in the wax with a stirring stick because the wax will turn into solid. Pour this liquid wax in the container immediately before it turns into solid. It may take almost 30 minutes to let it cool.

Just rub your finger on the surface of wax and apply it behind your ears and in your wrists.

Recipe 21: Jasmine Solid Perfume

- Beeswax: 1 tablespoon

- Almond oil: 1 tablespoon

- Glass container: 1

- Straw: 1

- Pyrex bowl or glass jar for mixing: 1

- Saucepan: 1

- Jasmine EO: 5 drops

- Rose EO: 4 drops

- Ylang-ylang EO: 2 drops

- Cedar EO: 2 drops

Directions:

Collect ingredients and supplies before starting you work. Measure out almond oil and wax in the glass jar. Put one inch water in a saucepan and place the bowl or jar containing wax in this water. Let this water boil to gradually melt wax.

Once the wax turn into liquid, you can remove it from heat. Mix in essential oils in the wax with a stirring stick because the wax will turn into solid. Pour this liquid wax in the container immediately before it turns into solid. It may take almost 30 minutes to let it cool.

Just rub your finger on the surface of wax and apply it behind your ears and in your wrists.

Recipe 22: Loveswept Solid Bar

- Almond oil: 2 tablespoons

- Beeswax: 2 tablespoons

- Jasmine EO: 2 to 4 drops

- Clove EO: 2 drops

- Vanilla Extract: 2 drops

Directions:

Collect ingredients and supplies before starting you work. Measure out almond oil and wax in the glass jar. Put one inch water in a saucepan and place the bowl or jar containing wax in this water. Let this water boil to gradually melt wax.

Once the wax turn into liquid, you can remove it from heat. Mix in essential oils in the wax with a stirring stick because the wax will turn into solid. Pour this liquid wax in the container Immediately before it turns into solid. It may take almost 30 minutes to let it cool.

Just rub your finger on the surface of wax and apply it behind your ears and in your wrists.

Recipe 23: Sandalwood Perfume

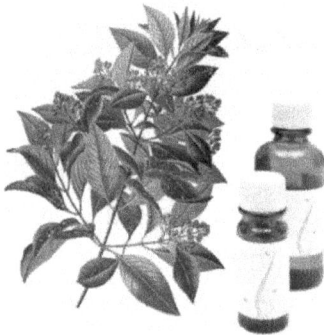

- Beeswax: 1 tablespoon
- Almond oil: 1 tablespoon
- Glass container: 1
- Straw: 1

- Pyrex bowl or glass jar for mixing: 1

- Saucepan: 1

- Jasmine EO: 5 drops

- Rose EO: 4 drops

- Sandalwood EO: 2 drops

- Cedar EO: 2 drops

Directions:

Collect ingredients and supplies before starting you work. Measure out almond oil and wax in the glass jar. Put one inch water in a saucepan and place the bowl or jar containing wax in this water. Let this water boil to gradually melt wax.

Once the wax turn into liquid, you can remove it from heat. Mix in essential oils in the wax with a stirring stick because the wax will turn into solid. Pour this liquid wax in the container immediately before it turns into solid. It may take almost 30 minutes to let it cool.

Just rub your finger on the surface of wax and apply it behind your ears and in your wrists.

Recipe 24: Fruity Perfume

- 35 drops grapefruit EO

- 15 drops orange EO

- 1 tablespoon beeswax pastilles

- 10 drops Vetiver essential oil

- 5 drops roman chamomile EO

- 10 drops Clary Sage EO

Directions:

Collect ingredients and supplies before starting you work. Measure out almond oil and wax in the glass jar. Put one inch water in a saucepan and place the bowl or jar containing wax in this water. Let this water boil to gradually melt wax.

Once the wax turn into liquid, you can remove it from heat. Mix in essential oils in the wax with a stirring stick because the wax will turn into solid. Pour this liquid wax in the container immediately before it turns into solid. It may take almost 30 minutes to let it cool.

Just rub your finger on the surface of wax and apply it behind your ears and in your wrists.

Recipe 25: Earthen Scent

- 20 drops lavender EO

- 14 drops cedarwood EO

- 1 tablespoon beeswax pastilles

- 30 drops marjoram essential oil

- 3 drops ylang-ylang EO

Direction:

Use microwave or double boiler to melt the beeswax. It is time to mix all essential oils in the beeswax. You have to pour this mixture in one jar or bottle. It is easy to pour solid perfume in a heart-shaped or round locket to keep it always with you.

Chapter 8: Amazing All-Natural Perfumes

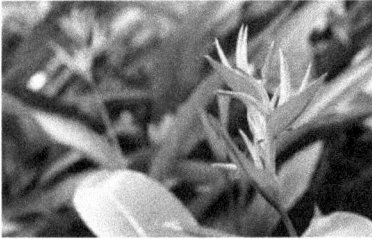

If you want natural perfumes with unique ingredients, you can get the advantage of these recipes.

Recipe 26: Chocolate Scented Blend

- Water (distilled): 2 cups

- Perpetual essential oil: 5 drops

- 100 Proof vodka: 3 tablespoons

- Vanilla EO: 10 drops

- Cocoa EO: 10 drops

Directions:

In the first step, add vodka (if using) in one jar and put all the ingredients and shake them well. It will be good to secure this mixture in a dark bottle and put this bottle in one dark and cold place for almost seven days. You can rub it on your pulse points to enjoy the enduring fragrance.

Recipe 27: Lemon and Orange Blend

- 2 cups water (distilled)
- 5 drops perpetual essential oil
- 3 tablespoons 100 Proof vodka
- 10 drops Orange EO
- 10 drops Lemon EO

Directions:

In the first step, add vodka (if using) in one jar and put all the ingredients and shake them well. It will be good to secure this mixture in a dark bottle and put this bottle in one dark and cold place for almost seven days. You can rub it on your pulse points to enjoy the enduring fragrance.

Recipe 28: Peppermint and Lemon Blend

- 2 cups water (distilled)

- 5 drops peppermint essential oil

- 3 tablespoons 100 Proof vodka (Optional)

- 10 drops sandalwood EO

- 10 drops Rose EO

Directions:

In the first step, add vodka (if using) in one jar and put all the ingredients and shake them well. It will be good to secure this mixture in a dark bottle and put this bottle in one dark and cold place for almost seven days. You can rub it on your pulse points to enjoy the enduring fragrance.

Recipe 29: Apricot Perfume

- 2 cups water (distilled)

- 5 drops perpetual essential oil

- 3 tablespoons Almond oil or Vodka

- 10 drops apricot EO

- 10 drops Sandalwood EO

Directions:

In the first step, add vodka (if using) in one jar and put all the ingredients and shake them well. It will be good to secure this mixture in a dark bottle and put this bottle in one dark and cold place for almost seven days. You can rub it on your pulse points to enjoy the enduring fragrance.

Recipe 30: Cinnamon Perfume

- Water (distilled): 2 cups

- Cinnamon essential oil: 5 drops

- 100 Proof vodka or Almond Oil: 3 tablespoons

- Sandalwood EO: 10 drops

- Neem EO: 10 drops

Directions:

In the first step, add vodka (if using) in one jar and put all the ingredients and shake them well. It will be good to secure this mixture in a dark bottle and put this bottle in one dark and cold place for almost

seven days. You can rub it on your pulse points to enjoy the enduring fragrance.

Chapter 9: Deodorant Recipes

If you want to make deodorant or body spray, you can get the advantage of these recipes. Get the advantage of these recipes:

Recipe 31: DIY Deodorant

• Coconut oil: ½ cup

• Baking soda: ½ cup

• Essential oils of your choice: 40 to 60 drops

Directions:

Mix in coconut oil and baking soda in one bowl along with essential oils. Store this deodorant in a glass jar and use as per your needs.

Recipe 32: Citrus Body Spray

• 15 Drops Grapefruit EO

• 5 drops of Lavender EO

- 8 Ounces distilled Water

- 1 tablespoon Hazel

Directions:

In the first step, add vodka (if using) in one jar and put all the ingredients and shake them well. It will be good to secure this mixture in a dark bottle and put this bottle in one dark and cold place for almost seven days. You can rub it on your pulse points to enjoy the enduring fragrance.

Recipe 33: Comfort Your Body

- Distilled Water: 8 Ounces

- Hazel: 1 tablespoon

- Cinnamon leaf EO: 10 drops

- Sweet orange EO: 15 drops

Directions:

In the first step, add vodka (if using) in one jar and put all the ingredients and shake them well. It will be good to secure this mixture in a dark bottle and put this bottle in one dark and cold place for almost

seven days. You can rub it on your pulse points to enjoy the enduring fragrance.

Recipe 34: Body Spray to Empower Your Brain

- Distilled Water: 8 Ounces

- Hazel: 1 tablespoon

- Rosemary oil: 5 drops

- Patchouli oil: 10 drops

- Peppermint oil: 10 drops

Directions:

In the first step, take one jar and put all the ingredients and shake them well. It will be good to secure this mixture in a dark bottle and put this bottle in one dark and cold place for almost seven days. You can rub it on your pulse points to enjoy the enduring fragrance.

Recipe 35: Jasmine Deodorant

- Distilled water: 1 tablespoon

- Vodka: 2 tablespoons

Jasmine blend

- Lavender: 5 drops

- Jasmine: 30 drops

- Vanilla: 5 drops

Directions:

In the first step, add vodka (if using) in one jar and put all the ingredients and shake them well. It will be good to secure this mixture in a dark bottle and put this bottle in one dark and cold place for almost seven days. You can rub it on your pulse points to enjoy the enduring fragrance.

Chapter 10: Precautions To Use Essential Oil Perfumes

Essential oils and their perfumes are good for your skin. There are a few oils that should be used with special precautions. For your assistance, there is some guidance:

• There is no need to leave these oils in extreme temperatures, such as a freezer, hot cars, and near windows.

• Keep essential oils away from direct sunlight.

• Some essential oils can break down any plastic bottle; therefore, you shouldn't store them in plastic containers.

• It will be bad to keep the bottles of essential oils open because oxidation process can affect the potency of oil.

• There is no need to heat or boil your oils to allocate them aromatically. They can lose their therapeutic value.

• There is no need to use oils in the hot tub.

• Always use diluted essential oils because undiluted oils can irritate your skin.

• There is no reason to expose your skin to photosensitive oils before going out to the sun. After applying these oils to your skin, you should keep yourself away from the sun for almost 12 hours. All citrus oils are photosensitive oils.

• These oils are not good to put in your nose, eyes, and ears. If the essential oil accidently goes into your eyes, there is no need to use water to wash your eyes. It can increase your pain and chances of damage. You can use a carrier oil to draw any oil out of your eyes. You can also use a cotton cloth to clean oil from your eyes.

• If you are uncomfortable with any oil, you should avoid their use. There should search reliable oils by your sensitive skins and allergies.

• There is no need to give empty bottles of essential oils to your children to play. The residue of these oils will be there in the bottles; you should handle with care.

• You should be careful by using oils after and before bath and swimming. Sometimes, use of essential oils after taking a bath can cause clogging in open pores. The water may drive oil into your skin.

It is essential to keep these oils away from your pets and children. After coming out of tanning both, you should stay away from the sun for almost six hours after treatment. Essential oils have flammable qualities; hence, you should keep them away from fire, candles, gas cookers, matches, and cigarettes. You can test these oils on a small part of your skin to check allergies.

You can use fresh rose petals to diffuse them in base oils and mix essential oils in this diffused blend. There are various choices for you to make organic blends. It is time to get rid of ordinary perfumes full of chemicals. You can use recipes given in this book to make healthy combinations. These are equally good to send as a gift.

Organic perfumes require the use of essential oils, rose water and fruit extracts. You can buy your favorite ingredients from the market. Homemade perfumes are safe for your environment, and you can use them without any health problem. It is possible to make your dream fragrance and send it as a gift to your friends and impress them. If you want to send something unique, you can follow the recipes given in this book. There are lots of fragrances that you can use on different occasions. You can prepare a personalized fragrance for your wedding. It will be a good way to improve your overall health.

Chapter 11: Homemade / Organic Perfumes Versus Synthetic Perfumes

Perfumes are well-loved by many and in some circumstances, even considered to be luxuries that people indulge in. However, were you aware of the fact that some of these bottled fragrances actually contain chemicals that can be quite toxic to the body? This is the truth that not a lot of perfume lovers are aware of. In fact, about 95% of the chemicals used in some of the most popular scents were actually derived from petroleum.

This is one of the reasons why there are people who are allergic to it. It can trigger asthma, rashes and a few other illnesses if used wrongly.

If you think that perfumes are made of ingredients of the flowers and plants they are suppose to smell of - be skeptical. Lilies' scent may not have the same floral essences as it. The majority of contemporary perfumes are made of synthetic materials and their scents are made from petroleum distillates. Why? It is because the use of synthetic ingredients has greatly assisted in the expansion of a perfumer's repertoire of scents they could choose from.

The perfumes were also less expensive to make which allowed a wider range of people to take pleasure in the scent. Raw materials can be costly and popular scents are the most expensive, such as ambergris, musk and the rare plants that were popular at the time.

The advancement of perfume manufacturing has meant that perfumes could be recreated in a lab with the help of the byproducts (such like coal tar) produced during the Industrial Revolution. This also allowed perfumers to create scents that were not in a position to bottle previously for example, lily and Lilac.

The studies conducted by the EPA have revealed that a lot of modern perfumes may contain hazardous chemicals, such as acetone the benzaldehyde compound, benzyl alcohol camphor, benzyl alcohol and ethyl acetate. They also contain the limonene, linalool, ethanol and Methylene chloride. When inhaled, these substances could cause:

* Various central nervous system disorders

* Nausea

* Speech slurred

* Dizziness

* Drool

* Eye irritation and throat, mouth, the skin and lungs

* Headaches

* Kidney damage

* Ataxia

* Respiratory failure

* Fatigue

In a separate study, two different types of dangerous chemicals were identified as common components in a variety of perfumes, regardless of the brand. These include synthetic musks and phthalates. Consider it this way. Because perfumes are sprayed directly to the skin, continuous exposure, as well as the relative amount we consume, can significantly contribute to the onset of the adverse side effects caused through these substances. That's why we must be cautious when it comes to choosing the right fragrance for us. We're not only risking our health but also in danger of exposing our loved ones the same dangers.

Why should you choose natural?

There are, thankfully, completely natural and safe alternatives to synthetic perfumes. Natural perfumes, as their name suggests, only utilize organic materials which are all from nature. When you use these scents there is no need to be concerned about the various chemicals listed above and the negative effects they could be having on your body. They do not contain anything the EPA doesn't approve of, even though they are made from natural substances. It is safe to say that you can be assured that they'll work and in harmony with your body and won't cause any health problems even if you are using frequently or for extended times.

Synthetic ingredients can be more expensive however they're not superior - at least not for our health, nor the scents we purchase. Take it in this manner natural ingredients possess more vitality and a sense of being. In spite of the method of preparation some of these ingredients contain specific ingredients and substances that improve our skin. Certain ingredients even offer scent benefits that are believed to relax the body and mind. With no harsh chemicals, perfumes have a greener outlook. This is good news since whenever we apply these products our air and the surrounding environment is also affected directly. Chemicals can affect the quality of the air and, in turn, impact us too. When you purchase something that is all natural that is organic, you will receive the best of nature's gift in its most natural form. What's more wonderful than this?

Why is it important to stay clear of synthetic perfume?

Around 60% of the stuff you apply to your skin is absorbed into the bloodstream. While your skin may be the most important organ of the body, it doesn't have filters like the liver and kidneys of our body. The skin is responsible for all the filtering itself. Take into consideration that around 95 percent of the chemicals that are found in the commercial fragrances have synthetics that are made from petroleum and natural gas and petrochemicals. They are absorbed by the skin and then into the bloodstream. They could then act as a catalyst for various health problems and skin-related ailments.

The skin can absorb these chemicals by direct application through spraying or rub the scent directly onto it, or through exposure to scents that are sprayed into the air by anyone around you. For certain people, the impact is usually instantaneous, particularly when they are sensitive to the substances the perfume could contain. From a simple sneeze to severe allergic reactions, the negative effects of perfume are many. For women who are pregnant it is crucial that they avoid the use of artificial fragrances. This is for their personal health and the baby's.

Unfortunately, to safeguard the trade secrets of their brands, the perfume manufacturers actually have the permission of FDA to hide information about the ingredients in their perfumes and therefore, you can't completely believe what the label is telling you. There might be dangerous chemical compounds in it that aren't listed on the bottle's label. What exactly does this mean? It basically permits companies to incorporate all kinds of chemicals into their products. Sensitizers and other hormone disruptors are but one of the many.

Some of the most discussed substances that consumers ought to be aware of are:

Parabens are chemical preservatives commonly found in commercial scents. They can affect the release and production of hormones within the body.

Phthalates A different popular preservative for fragrances, look out for that many perfumes sold in the market contain high concentrations of this. Unbeknownst to many, it's carcinogen, and can cause many health problems if employed for a long period of time. It could cause liver and kidney damage as well as cause birth problems during pregnancy, and decrease the sperm count of men and lead to early breast growth.

Synthetic Musks - Do you love the smell of musks? If your perfume is made with synthetic musks in its creation you might consider rethinking your decision to go to another bottle. There are studies that show several kinds of synthetic musks which can disrupt hormones. The research is ongoing to determine the harm it may do to the body. However, there is evidence to suggest that it has adverse effect if used continuously.

Why are natural fragrances so costly?

Natural scents are typically more expensive, primarily due to the ingredients used to make they are more costly as compared to synthetic versions. A lot of natural scents are made of natural extracts from nature which are difficult to find. As an example the price of rose oil is about 500 for each ounce and is predicted to increase again in the coming year. For the cost however, you'll get an aroma that is truly divine and you do not have to be concerned about its effects on your health. Natural perfumes are also known to have more fragrance they are compared to synthetic perfumes.

The Essentials of Creating Perfumes

There are numerous kinds of perfumes on the market, however how they're made generally follows the same principle. If you're considering making your own at home, these are the essential things to be aware of.

It is crucial to be aware that the composition of fragrances is based on the pyramid. The base notes comprise the majority of the fragrance and therefore, it is the most prominent. To assist you in understanding this more this is a short overview of the meanings of these notes and how they affect the way perfumes smell:

The top notes make up only a small portion of the scent. It's what you detect when you take the bottle out of the box or when you first apply the fragrance. These notes don't stay as long as other scents and are usually rather light when you first smell them.

Middle notes which are also known as heart notes comprise between 30 and 40 percent of overall scent. It becomes more apparent when the fragrance's top note has was gone. They're longer in duration than top notes, but it eventually fades also.

As we've discussed earlier, make up the largest proportion of the overall scent. It's the longest-lasting of the notes. It doesn't typically show up until after what's known by"the "drydown" or when it has completely disappeared.

Commonly used scents for every note:

The top notes are cardamom clary sage, coriander, basil, grapefruit Eucalyptus, lavender lemon, juniper mandarin, peppermint pine, neroli, petigrain, thyme, and tea tree.

Middle Notes or Heart notes: Cinnamon Cedar wood, Geranium clove, jasmine, marjoram Palm rose, frankincense rose, chamomile rose and ylang ylang.

Top or Base notes Patchouli vanilla, benzoin and vetiver.

Blending Tips:

The first thing to think about is the note of the oil as well as the other types they might mix well with. To do this, some studies is required. There are many aromatherapy books on the market both on the internet and offline, so obtaining the data you require will be simple. Like everything else it will always be some trial and failure.

First, decide on the note of the heart you'd like to use. It is helpful to be certain from the beginning of your research about the fragrance you want to create. Knowing this will help you to pick the appropriate essential oils to achieve the desired effect. Take into consideration the mood you'd like to create, the type of look the fragrance will have and also the age range you intend to target. If you're creating gender-specific scents, you should consider the type of scent that works well with both female and male customers.

Second: Choose the base note. It could be a combination comprising two or three oils. Regardless, take note of this. One of the most effective methods to determine which scents are a perfect match for your heart note is to perform an experiment with strips. This means you'll require strips of paper which you can place the scents you prefer. Combine them and determine what scents complement each to create an harmonious mixture of scents that is not overwhelming.

It is also possible to use tops of bottles. You can hold them in a row and go through the air or with your nose to see whether they blend well. It's a process that requires manual effort however, it definitely works. A little practice is required Of course however, if you practice it often, you'll get the "perfumer's scent". Keep a notepad as well! This will help to refer to in the future if you need to recreate specific combinations again.

Third: After the second step is completed it is possible to add the note of your choice to the chosen base note. Be aware that you can't alter this portion. Base should sit on the lower part like the name suggests. The middle note or the heart should be at the middle.

Fourth: Finally, you can finish the entire fragrance with your preferred top note. Make sure that it's in sync with the other notes you've added to allow the scent to be cohesive to it. It isn't advisable to randomly mix up notes since it can cause the fragrance smell overwhelming or even overwhelming.

Final: After you have added all of your notes, the final thing to do is add the modification.

Modifiers are another scent that is added to scents to create a distinctive scent. Modifiers should be used in a limited amount, usually just a little. If you smell the modifier you applied, it's a sign that you've used too many. You can reduce the amount by increasing your heart rate. However, be cautious when applying it since it can change the smell that you've worked so hard on.

When mixing oils, begin by using just three or two. If you'd prefer to keep it basic and easy, choose to use one oil to create your entire scent. It is easy to tell if the scent is balanced by sniffing it. If you are unable to identify any of its elements, but you can still detect the fruitiness or woodiness that you desired, then you were successful in creating a balanced scent. Take into consideration that scents change older they get. The top middle and bottom notes are more apparent with time however the overall scent will remain the same.

Scent Classifications

Have you been aware of the various ways people talk about certain fragrances? With regards to this there are a variety of types of classifications that are used to identify the kind of scent you're creating. It's all based upon the components you've chosen and which ones you've chosen to create each note. Here are some illustrations to comprehend the basics better:

"Citrus scents": They are usually created from essential oils like orange, bergamot and lemon. They're refreshing scents, but they're also light than other scents, and are often used in top notes. However, this causes them to be very volatile and they do not last for long, when compared to other scents.

"Refreshing Scents": They are generally soothing and pleasant to the nose. They also smell clean, fresh and crisp However, it all depends on the blend you choose to use in your scent. In contrast to citrus scents they tend to have a stronger fragrance and are commonly employed to cover the base notes that can be quite intense. They can balance that out.

* Herbaceous scents: Like the citrus scents, they typically smell fresh and clear. But, it's more of a green scent. The smell of greenery. They are a bit diffusive and could be popular top notes since they appeal to many people.

* Floral scents: Floral notes are considered to be the most varied , and are typically used to create feminine scents due to their softness and softness their scents. There are however, some which can be strong scents and are usually blended with other florals. Many people wear single notes of

flowers in small quantities and also as separated if they are needed. But, many believe that choosing the right mix will bring out particular characteristics of the note and add more weight.

* Oriental Scents: Oriental notes are those made from ingredients usually sourced in sources in Far East. They include more spicier notes like Vanilla and sandalwood, as well as the frankincense. They are typically the longest-lasting and provide fragrances with a deeper smell and a warmness that other oils can't provide.

Organic Perfume Recipes that you can make at home

We've already learned the importance of staying clear of commercial perfumes because they contain toxic chemicals that can harm our bodies and health through long-term exposure. We also have established that there are alternatives available, natural fragrances that utilize the natural ingredients that nature has to offer. But, they can be expensive in a specialty retailer.

This is a natural fact because the ingredients used in perfumes tend to cost higher than synthetic ones. In case this sounds like something that you're not a fan of There is another alternative and that is making your own perfumes from your home.

You've learned the fundamentals of mixing in the previous chapter, so this time, we'll concentrate on recipes that are simple to replicate that will allow you to start experimenting. Make sure that if it's your first time creating scents, you must always take guidelines for safety and leave plenty of room for errors. There will always be trials and error to get familiar with the process. The most important thing is to be creative and to enjoy your work!

Jasmine Perfume

In the traditional and natural medical field, Jasmine is typically used to alleviate anxiety and nerves. Although it continues to work to treat these conditions but it is more well recognized for its ethereal scent it produces. it.

A floral scent, but not overwhelming, this flower can give any fragrance a warm and more sensual feel to it. A scent that will surely aid in relaxation. Vanilla oil is added to aid by calming the fragrance and helps it last longer. The lavender is intended to help bridge the two.

Ingredients:

* 2 tbsp. of vodka

* 1 tbsp. orange blossom water. It is also possible to use the water that is distilled.

* Jasmine blend

* 30 drops jasmine

* 5 drops lavender

* 5 drops vanilla

Directions:

Mix the essential oil blend with vodka and let it sit for at minimum a few days. After that you should add your distillate water or orange blossom water, and shake it vigorously. Let it sit for at least 4 weeks in a cool, dark part of your house. If you notice any sediments forming, you can clean it off with cheesecloth and then transfer the scent into a new bottle.

Vanilla Oil Perfume

To make this recipe, you'll require some patience since it takes a while before you are able to utilize the recipe. It's all worth it however it produces an aroma of vanilla which is durable. It can be used in a variety of ways too. It can be used for body scents or bath oil, or even as a freshener for your room. The best part? It's natural, which means you don't need to worry about unwelcome adverse consequences.

Ingredients:

* 8-10 vanilla beans

* Jojoba or Almond Oil

* Vodka

Directions:

* Cut about 8-10 parts of vanilla beans, then cut the beans in half with an instrument. They don't need to be expensive or costly and you do not need to shell out a large amount of money to purchase it. Then, you can take beans and put it in the small container. After you've scraped the entire mess then cut the beans and put them in the container, too.

Add enough vodka to completely cover the contents of the container. The vodka will absorb inside the coffee beans, and take in their vanilla aroma. Be sure to not overdo it because it can affect the final scent.

* Then, remove the jar and store it somewhere dry and not freezing. Let it sit for three to two months, based on the intensity of the scent that you'd like to use. You can monitor the development through opening your jar each once a day and checking the smell to determine how absorption is progressing. It is recommended to choose a dark-colored container for this purpose and be sure that the blend isn't in direct sunlight since this could alter the results.

Once the mixture is done you can make use of a fine strainer, like cheesecloth or cotton, to strain the liquid. This should allow you to eliminate any solid pieces, and only extract the essential liquid to create the scent. Transfer the fragrance to a different container and add the oil from Jojoba. You should use about double what amount you compare it to liquid. You can use your vanilla beans and paste to make an additional batch of scent. It might not be as powerful as the original however it will be as effective. If you're looking for the same strength it is merely adding additional beans to the mix.

* To help your perfume last longer, keep it in a cool, dry area.

Citrus Perfume

If you're in search of an amazing, light scent take a look at this citrus-based concoction. It can also be used as an aromatherapy productthat refreshes the senses by delivering a refreshing aroma. You can use it to scent your linens, your house or clothes, and every other space in your home that needs an extra increase in scent.

Ingredients:

* 1 tbsp. of Jojoba oil

* 2 tbsps. in pure alcohol or vodka

• 30 drops essential oils that are citrusy. It is recommended to use Grapefruit, Sweet Orange lavender and peppermint.

* 1 tbsp. of distillated water

Directions:

Start by adding Jojoba oil into the container. Check that it's free of dirt before you pour any substance into it. Then, you can you can add your alcohol.

Then, follow up by adding essential oils in the following order:

1. Base Note - 10 drops the grapefruit

2. Middle Note: 10 drops of Sweet Orange essential oil and 5 drops of peppermint essential oil

3. Top Note: five drops of the lavender blend. If you don't own a blend or prefer not to make use of one, any lavender essential oil can perform just as well.

* Mix some distilled water in the dropper.

Be sure that you thoroughly mix it before placing it in an opaque glass container. It can be stored for up to 48 hours , or even up to 6 weeks, regardless of how powerful you would like the fragrance to be. Be aware that the longer you allow it to remain, the stronger the scent will become.

* Once it is ready to filter, transfer it to a different bottle.

Lavender Scented Solid Perfume

The majority of people know the advantages of lavender. It is among the most well-known essential oils due to the fact that it is used in a variety of ways. It is a good idea to keep a small bottle it in your pocket can provide a natural remedy for various ailments, including headaches and jetlag. As a scent, it is soothing and light. It's possible that you will feel all tensions disappearing when you rub it on. You can use it as a sleep aid by gently rub your wrists before you go to sleep in the evening. It will aid you in falling asleep faster and more comfortably.

Ingredients:

* 1 tbsp. of beeswax grated

* 1 tbsp. of almond oil

* 5-6 drops of lavender essential oil

Directions:

Mix the beeswax and almond oil together. Warm them gently until they both melt. You can do this using the microwave or stovetop with a low flame to accomplish this. Take care to adhere to the appropriate precautions when performing the procedure.

Once the mixture has been melted, stir the mixture before adding the lavender oil. After that, pour the mixture into a container that has a an easily fitting lid. Then let it sit or store it in the refrigerator to for it to set faster.

Once it has cured and you'll end up with something that looks like the consistency of a lotion. To useit, simply apply a tiny amount of it on the pulse points.

Herbal Garden Perfume

Do you want something more earthy? Then this will be the perfect recipe. It is made up of ingredients well-known for their ease on the body, this herbal fragrance is intended to be worn in any time of year. It's a deep scent in its fragrance and, depending on your preference it can be made with varying levels of richness.

Ingredients:

* 12-20 drops of Cedar wood, Vetiver Vanilla, Ylang Ylang, and Sandalwood.

* 1 tsp. of vanilla extract (optional)

* 25-30 drops of similar to Rose, Chamomile, Lavender or Geranium.

Amount of 12 to 15 drops Bergamot, Neroli or Wild Orange.

Four ounces alcohol are needed to keep scents intact and blend them. Spiced Rum is suggested for this to add a touch of depth to the scent you're making. You can, however, choose vodka or any other alcohol you like.

Directions:

Mix all of your oils based on which are your middle notes, top notes, and base notes. Be aware that this order is crucial and could alter the scent you're looking for in the wrong way. Allow the mix to remain inside the bottle over a couple of days, allowing it to mix.

Once you've got the aroma you desire Add your alcohol.

Shake well and store it in a dark, cool place in your home for a minimum of weeks or a month. This will allow the alcohol smell time to diminish and allow the scent from the oil to grow further.

Forms of Perfume

As there are a vast array of fragrances available fragrances are also diverse in the packaging they are available in and. The scent they emit is influenced by the length of time that a certain kind of scent can last. It's recommended to get familiar with the various options available. This is particularly important when you plan to create your own at home.

1. Perfumes based on water and alcohol

To do this, you will require vodka, oil, and distilled water. It is essential to have essential oils, too. Mix at least three distinct scents to create your top and middle notes. This requires some trial and error, so make sure you allow yourself plenty of time to study which scents work best one another. When you've found a combination that you are happy with note down the ingredients you used prior to reduce it using water/carrier oil.

2. Solid Perfume

They're great for the convenience as well as for their longevity. They are typically made from beeswax, oil and the option of essential oils blends. The most difficult part of making them is making sure the consistency is consistent. For newbies, this may be a difficult task but a lot of practice and testing will assist with this. Make sure it's difficult enough to stop the perfume from melting away and turning into a cream instead.

It is possible to add glitter to this particular kind of fragrance so that every time you apply it to your face, it contributes to the gorgeous glowing effect. It is best to keep them out of direct sunlight but if you are able to find the right proportion of your ingredients, you can create a scent that you can keep in your purse. The possibilities are endless for the kinds of scents that you can make using these ingredients, so let your imagination shine.

3. Spray or roll for oil on the body or on

This is a top choice among many perfume makers since it's easy to create and the components are readily available. Another advantage is that perfume oils are also known to be moisturizing for the skin due to the fact that they make usage of organic oils, such as jojoba , which is believed to be extremely nourishing. When it comes to wearing it, it's quite durable when compared to the alcohol-based or water-based fragrances. But, the body oils have a shorter shelf-life , and must be stored in a proper manner for them to last.

In terms of the scent it depends on the length of time the fragrance was allowed to remain" it may be strong and sultry. The majority of the time it is used with plants with aromatherapy properties in the formulation of perfume oils. But, you don't need to be restricted to these components alone.

4. Botanic Infused Cologne

Colognes that are lighter than perfumes are just as simple and enjoyable to make. The most appealing part is you could utilize real botanicals and herbs for making a scent that's yours to create. Some people prefer fresh flowers and herbs for their perfumes, which makes the scent a little less intense than if they use dried flowers. It's also possible to make a blend that is a mix of both, provided you follow the correct method for making the blend. Certain blends mix botanicals and herbs for example, vanilla and lavender.

In general, these colognes need to be allowed to sit for a minimum of weeks, however you may choose to reduce the time frame when you think you've attained the scent you desire. Be aware that the longer these blends set in the air, the more concentrated and sophisticated the scent will become. If you're looking to create different scents, include essential oils into the mix, too. Colognes might not last as long like perfumes, but they will certainly smell beautiful.

5. Talcum Perfume

The scent of scented talc is definitely not new, however, a most people are unaware that it could be used for perfumes as well. It's all about the composition as typical powders disappear in a matter of minutes and, if purchased from a commercial source they may have the same chemicals that are harmful as those that we have discussed previously. They are simple DIY however, so do not be concerned about it. To begin you'll need simple Talc powder. It is made of mineral talc, which can be typically discovered in metamorphic rocks.

It's completely natural, naturally and you'd like to preserve it as such.

Do not add perfumes purchased from stores to your perfume as it could alter the composition. Instead, you can use essential oils that are natural to create the fragrance you desire. Many people add the scent with fresh or dried plants mixed into the Talc. If the powder is allowed to sit for a set duration the powder will become the scent of the flowers it was mixed with.

The only thing be wary of is that certain individuals are allergic to the talc. It is important to do an allergy test on your skin before applying the powder over your body. They might not last as long as other scents however it will smell like a good perfume and can use it for a long period of time.

Chapter 12: Top Organic Perfumes

Did you know that a whiff of aroma can reduce pressure, improve your mood, and reduce tension in your muscles? In fact, it has been proven that the smells we surround us with constantly greatly affect our mental health (1). Are you looking to feel provocative but certain? Do you want to feel relaxed and peaceful? Refreshed and positive? Are you struggling to recall your favourite climbing route while working? Simply apply the right scent and take a long breath at any time you require a jolting beverage

In the event that you're in the market for a change to the quality of your fragrance, you should have the chance to add an aroma that is distinctive to the mix. The typical scents harness the power of real plant characteristics to create appealing, stimulating and valid scents. In this short guide for general scents I'll explain everything you need to know about common scents, including how they're created, the types of distinctive scents, as well as our list of the most natural scents tested by our experts in magnificence.

What is the process of making natural perfume?

The regular fragrance is produced by segregating the characters, waxes and oils from the plant-based fixings making use of two methods that include the CO_2 method (pressurized carbon dioxide used to eliminate phytochemicals from plant components) and the more direct approach (a specific dissolvable is employed to remove the oil extracted from in the plants). Both strategies are able to remove the most intense aroma with a secure method.

The most natural scents effortlessly blend novel, unique and captivating essential oils with the addition of concentrates into their formulas. The most memorable scents include jasmine flowers and rose otto, cedar wood, orange blossom tobacco, vetiver, vanilla and Neroli.

Once the embodiments have been eliminated, the scents are then mixed with regular alcohols, waxes or oils based on the kind of scent being produced.

Types OF NATURAL Perfumes

*Spray Perfumes Traditional fog or splash scents are typically made using natural liquor as their base. Natural liquor is incredibly dissolvable shower fragrance.

*Roll Ons and Oil Perfumes The essential oils are often combined with non-scented carrier oil (such like sunflower oil) to create a heightened regular oil scent. The fragrances can be brushed to the skin easily or applied using a roll onto a ball.

*Perfume Balms and solid Perfumes The majority of the fragrances are made by combining essential oils and plant extracts using a wax to create an intense scent. Simply apply these aroma with your fingers, just as you would apply a lip emollient.

Is ALCOHOL SAFE?

Regarding alcohol, you could be shocked to discover that scents containing liquor don't have to be a bad thing. Natural alcohols are an effect of the oil-making process. Many conventional perfumeries employ natural liquor as an place to store their fragrance. Liquor is used in scents to aid in bonding and combining the fixings, but it disappears quickly upon contact with skin, leaving only the pleasant fixings.

What is the best way to shop for natural perfumes?

The most effective method to verify if the scent is truly distinctive is to read the name of the scent. It is not like other types of names of magnificence authentically distinctive scents must be simple to identify. In the first place, you'll have to find simple normal, common, and natural fixings like CO_2 separates and absolutes, alcohol, basic oils (for instance, wine liquor) beeswax, plants that are extricated (amber pitch, amber, and the like.).

When it comes to fixings to avoid, take care to stay clear from the phthalates (generally simply referred to as "perfume" as well as "scent" in the mark of fixing). Phthalates were found to disrupt the endocrine as well as conceptual structure (2). Diethylphthalate (DEP) is an particular normal phthalate that is disguised under "aroma" in aromas that are traditional (3).

Lucky for you, our expert experts scoured through the entire spectrum of everyday scents. We sat down, smelt and analyzed a variety of fragrances to come up with this list of the best. These scents are crafted of delicious natural fixings and possess scents that are undisputed. Like most of the top-rated lists, you do not have to worry about the presence of parabens, phthalatesand petrochemicals and natural oils and colors, engineered scents PEG mix or anything else from our list of restrictive fixings.

The BEST natural and ORGANIC Perfumes

Flip over any container you have within your bathroom and search for fragrance or scent. We guarantee you'll find it on every running list of each item you utilize It is a common feature within the home's most common products. Why? Because shoppers want their products to smell nice. The problem? The organizations don't have a legal obligation to discover what scent is made of in the sense that it's seen as restricting.

Of the possible 2,947 fixings identified from the International Fragrance Association (IFRA) Aroma blends typically contain around a hundred synthetic compounds, with the major portion of which are engineered according to an earlier report, emit the same amount of concoction fumes emanating from the oil discharges of vehicles. These volatile natural mixtures (VOCs) are able to interact to proteins within our bodies that may trigger sensitive reactions (counting breathing problems, headaches, facial pains, cerebral pains and asthma attacks).

Over time, it can lead to more severe long-term effects on our health.

A study that examined 37 products that had fragrances for customers and discovered that 42 of VOCs they released were classified as toxic or hazardous under U.S. government laws. Most likely the most dangerous fixations that are found under the name of aroma (or another related word, like scent) contain phthalates (hormone disruptors that are linked to conceptional birth defects in infants and young males) along with nonoxynols and octoxynols (additionally constant hormone disruptions).

In relation to the distinctive aromas Essential oils used for scents can be extremely beneficial to your skin, but they could also cause irritations and consequently considered harmful to your health at certain quantities. The way the oil is prepared also matters. Retailers scrutinize the amount and quality of the basic oils they sell in the premium products they sell to ensure security but it is vital to buyers to be aware of the risks of purchasing directly from traditional or free oil brands.

For instance, a report from a few years ago found potentially risky synthetic blends in 24 business essential oils tested. Despite the fact that essential oils were labeled "regular," "natural," or "unadulterated," they were extracted from their original form, weakened, or incorporated with petrochemicals, which could be inhaled within your skin or inhaled.

Our suggestion: Call the magnificence brands you like and ask for the list of fixings used in their scents, as well as the method of sourcing of essential oils. Are they able to claim that they are organic, and if so, do they claim they were produced in a manner that is sustainable? Cross each fixing with an outsider, such as The Environmental

Working Group. You can also go a step further and ask that the brands you like change their names with the intention that they include the bulk the scent fixants into their labeling going forward.

As you get to know more, be familiar with our 19 editors' favorite fragrances without phthalates beneath. They range from natural and normal to a little less sour than the ones you're currently using as well as some fragrances that break the rules by delivering all-encompassing fragrance fixing simplicity.

Chapter 13: Starting What You Should Be Aware Of

Many people have begun to appreciate the value of using organic products at home. Organic products seem to be the trend of the future. If you're looking to cut costs by making your own perfumes, these DIY Colognes will assist you in doing the same.

The price of essential oils is less expensive than costly fragrances that contain ingredients and chemicals that can't even be identified. The majority of perfumes by larger companies in the beauty industry don't even list all ingredients on the label or bottle.

A lot of these ingredients are made up of petroleum or are natural gas bases. Certain chemicals have been proven to cause cancer if they're often used.

Furthermore, some of these chemicals can be very harmful for babies and children.

The main question here is, why not create your own fragrances and perfumes? Organically, natural method appears to be more beneficial and healthier, not just for you, but also for your entire family too.

Methods to make perfumes

There are a variety of ways to make perfume , and we've included more than 30 recipe ideas in the book to help you to try. Certain recipes come with specific instructions, while with others, you combine all the ingredients. Here's a brief description of how perfume making is done.

A lot of people prefer to use an alcohol-based base for their perfume-making. If you want to include alcohol in your perfume, add one an ounce 100 proof Vodka in addition to your essential oils.

If you're not a fan of alcohol and prefer using all-natural or organic products, then you can opt for sweet almond oil, fractionated coconut oil or jojoba oil.

These are oils that are thin that complement the essential oils well.

The main ingredient is thought of as the basis of your perfume. It can be your first smell that you feel after taking the first sniff of your perfume.

There are other ingredients that are included in the perfumes you wear, that are thought of as to be a mid-note and an under note. The mid note is the first scent you'll smell.

A lot of perfumes use oils such as bay Black pepper, Fennel pine, juniper and rosemary as their middle notes. Basil as well as cinnamon, coriander lemon, grapefruit and sage are excellent oils to put on an upper note. When you start making diverse recipes, you'll soon be able to understand how these notes work by playing around with the aromas.

An important point to keep in mind when making use of essential oils, is that you make use of dark glass bottles or containers.

The oils break down plastic and you'll be left with an unpleasant smell. It is best to keep the perfume in a dry area and, once you've created them, be sure that you let them infuse for at minimum 48 hours.

The sun's rays can degrade essential oils and create unneeded heat to them. Therefore, it is essential to keep them in a dark area. The best benefit of essential oils is they do not expire or go bad, which means you are able to continue using the oils in your scents and diffusers for many years.

Where can you buy your ingredients?

There are several ingredients to make your perfume. The first is that you'll require glass bottles or roll-on bottles. There are many online businesses which sell glass bottles at a wholesale price and you can score a affordable price for a huge quantity. Companies such as Uline provide great bulk discounts.

You can also purchase glass bottles from firms like Michaels, Hobby Lobby, the

Container Store, ebottles.com, Amazon as well as Bed Bath and beyond.

When you have the number of bottles you require then it's time to get the neutral bases. If you'd like to make use of vodka, you can buy it at any liquor store within your region. If you'd like to use coconut oil , or sweet almond oil, there are several choices.

You can purchase all of these products from the following stores: Amazon, GNC, bulkapothocary.com, Vitamin Shoppe, Whole Foods and any other stores selling natural foods and herb shops within your local area.

Essential oils can be bought from a variety of locations. One of the most popular online retailers is doTERRA However, you can also purchase the oils at any natural food retailer. You can also purchase them in stores such as Walgreens, Whole Foods, Sprouts, Piping Rock, Young Living, and Eden's Garden.

Let's make perfumes!

Once you have an idea of the ingredients you'll require, we'll start to prepare the recipes. The recipes in this article can create very pleasant smells. If they don't have specific directions, they will follow this recipe.

The basic recipe:

One Ounce neutral-base (Sweet almond oil coconut oil, jojoba oil, or 100 Proof vodka)

Essential oils in drops

Place the neutral base inside the bottle made of glass first. Add the drops of oil to the glass bottle.

It is important to shake the bottle thoroughly. Place the lid on the bottle and keep it in a cool, dark location for at least 48 hours.

Once you master this basic recipe, you'll soon be creating the most popular scents at the convenience of your home without having to worry about the gas-based chemicals that will be leaking on your skin.

Seasonal Fragrances

Spring

The spring season is upon us:

If spring is in the air, emotions in people start to shirt. It is the season of the rebirth of many animals and numerous people.

There are many emotions that are that spring brings and these emotions can be incorporated into the perfumes you create. The emotions that arise with the change of seasons are happiness, serenity, love of hope, joy romantic, new beginnings. A lot of people believe that spring is the period of renewal and a chance to change their habits and lives.

There are a variety of scents connected with spring, and many of them are featured in fine perfumes created by companies selling their fragrances throughout the world.

It is possible to incorporate these scents in your personal scents. The scents you choose to wear will remind you of why you enjoy spring so much , and what emotions are evoked within your mind during this time of year. The most well-known scents that springtime perfumes can be found in include vanilla, lavender and jasmine. Also, rose and magnolia.

Mix of Fairies from the Forest

40 drops from sweet orange oils

20 drops of oil from cedar wood

10 drops of oil containing peppermint

5 drops of rosemary oil

Romance is in the Garden

20 drops from sweet essential oils of orange

5 drops of essential lavender oil

10 drops of essential oil patchouli

10 drops of essential oil for cedar wood

5 drops of ylang ylang essential oil

5 drops of Bergamot

A bit of romance

1 Tablespoon grape seed oil

1 tablespoon vodka

5 Drops of palmarosa essential oil

3 drops of rose essential oil

1 drop of essential rose geranium oil

1 drop of ylang ylang essential oil

Cucumber splash

1 Cucumber

1 Lemon squeeze

1 Teaspoon of Aloe Vera gel

1 Tablespoon rose water

Special instructions Peel the cucumber, then chop it into small pieces.

The cucumber is blended for around 1 minute. Remove the juice into the bowl. Then, add the other ingredients to the bowl. Mix it all together or dump everything into your blender for mixing it.

Young

1 tablespoon vodka

1 Tablespoon grape seed oil

9 drops of essential grapefruit oil

1 drop of essential oil rose geranium

1 Drop of ylang-ylang

In the garden

2 tablespoons of almond sweet oil

6 Tablespoons of premium vodka

2 Tablespoons (1/2 cup) of water from the spring

6 drops of essential oil for cedar wood

15 drops of essential clove oil

9 drops of essential lavender oil

Special instructions Special instructions: Add all the oils into an empty container and shake. Then , add vodka and almond oil and shake. The mixture should be left for at least at least 48 hours. If you prefer a stronger aroma then let it rest for about one week.

Spring flowers

4 Ounces of coconut oil fractionated

17 drops of ylang ylang essential oil

17 drops of essential oil blood orange

137

5 drops of lavender essential oil

Autumn

The leaves of autumn are starting to fall

The autumn season is a transitional one. Similar to spring it is a time of many emotions and emotions that are triggered when the leaves begin to change color from red to yellow.

There are many celebrations that occur during the fall months like Thanksgiving and Halloween. These holidays usually inspire us to decorate our homes with shades of browns, oranges and reds. This is the time of year when we begin to put on the warm clothing and scarves.

The autumn season also brings back many emotions and smells. Many people associate the season with being able to hold hands with their loved ones and experiencing the feeling of warmth and comfort. The changing leaves make some of us recall our childhoods, when we used to play in the leaves of the backyard.

The autumn season also offers outdoors activities such as hiking and camping. The changing colors of the leaves from the mountains isn't just stunning, but it is also extremely romantic.

Halloween is the season of the year that includes pumpkin carving and apple cider. Two distinct times in the fall that bring people joy.

The scents of autumn are extremely relaxing and warm. Pumpkin and apple cider are among the most popular scents that are enjoyed in the autumn season, however you can also add other scents to your perfumes to help keep in mind why you enjoy the crisp air and red leaves. Cinnamon, sageand vanilla, wild orange coriander and saffron are just a few scents that can be incorporated to your perfumes made from scratch.

In the Woods

10 drops of essential oil for cedar wood

20 drops of essential oil of frankincense

Autumn Leaves

30 drops of wild orange essential oil

30 drops of essential oil patchouli

10 drops of essential clove oil

Halloween

20 drops of essential oil of wild orange

20 drops of essential oil of frankincense

10 drops of essential cassia oil

Give Thanks

10 drops of essential ginger oil

10 drops of essential oil of cinnamon

20 drops of essential coriander oil

10 drops of essential oil of clove

It's autumn!

20 drops of essential oil cassia

20 drops of essential oil of wild orange

Oatmeal cookies

20 drops of essential oil for cedar wood

20 drops of essential oil cassia

30 drops of wild orange essential oil

Days of woodsiness

4 drops of essential oil of spruce

2 drops of needle of Fir essential oil

2 drops of essential oil from cedarwood

1 Drop of essential vetiver oil

1 drop of bergamot essential oil

1 Teaspoon Jojoba Oil

The Sirens

7 drops of essential oil sandalwood

14 drops of essential rose oil

9 drops from Bergamot essential oil

Mysterious

1 Tablespoon grape seed oil

1 tablespoon vodka

8 drops of essential oil sandalwood

3 drops of essential lavender oil

1 drop of essential oil for cedarwood

Summer

Summertime fun for everyone:

The summer season is among the most joyful and pleasant seasons of many people's lives.

The summer is when many people go on their holidays, so they think of this time as a time for beach and ocean. Also, they view the summer season as one of the freedom of being.

Many people also think of summer as rivers, parks Ice cream, and having fun with friends at the entire night. Summer brings about a lot of joy and pleasant feelings within people.

There are many popular summer scents which are included in a variety of perfume recipes. However, there are many that you can include that aren't mentioned here , like watermelon, sweet citrus, lime, orange lemon, grapefruit, honeysuckle and jasmine mango, strawberry, and. The scents for summer focus on upon warmer and fruity scents.

These scents will trigger memories from the sunshine and all its warmth.

I love the sun

20 drops of juniper berry essential oil

20 drops of essential grapefruit oil

10 drops of essential oil from wild orange

Simple Life

1 teaspoon of Jojoba oil

1 ounce of water

5 drops of essential oil jasmine

3 drops of oil from lemon

3 drops of oil in orange

3 drops of essential oil sandalwood

Grateful

20 drops of essential oil of clove

20 drops from sweet essential oils of orange

10 drops of Geranium essential oil

Real Love

20 drops of essential lavender oil

20 drops of ylang ylang essential oil

20 drops of essential oil of chamomile

10 drops of essential oil patchouli

Lavender vanilla

1 cup vodka

Two Tablespoons vegetable Glycerin

1 cup of dried lavender flower petals

2 Whole vanilla beans

15 drops of essential lavender oil

10 Drops of vanilla essential oil

Special instructions Special instructions: Cut the vanilla beans down to the smallest size you can and then place them along with lavender flowers, vodka and lavender in an glass jar. Let the mixture infuse for around one week. Then strain the ingredients and add the vegetable glycerin as well as essential oils. Allow this to infuse for 4 to six weeks. The aroma will become stronger depending on the length of time you'd like to let it infuse.

Vanilla mist

6 Cardamom seeds

1 Teaspoon pure vanilla extract

1 Cup water

Special instructions for the seeds: Bring them to a simmer with half a cups of water. Allow the ingredients to cool, then put them into the spray bottle. Mix in vanilla, shake and add.

Happy Day

7 drops of pine oil

14 drops of lemongrass oil

9 drops of sweet essential oil of orange

Luscious

1 tablespoon vodka

1 Tablespoon grapeseed oil

6 Drops of essential lavender oil

4 drops of essential oil of frankincense

1 drop of essential rose geranium oil

A bit of spice

1 tablespoon of vodka

1 Tablespoon grapeseed oil

8 drops of essential oil from sandalwood

2 drops of essential oil from wild orange

1 drop of essential oil patchouli

1 drop of ylang-ylang essential oil

Sweetie pie

1 tablespoon vodka

1 Tablespoon grapeseed oil

5 Drops of vanilla essential oil

4 Drops of cocoa Absolute

1 drop of ylang-ylang essential oil

Joyful

Half Teaspoons of Vanilla

1 1/2 Teaspoons of essential rose oil

4 drops of musk essential oil

15 drops of ambergris oil

15 drops of jasmine oil

4 drops of Neroli oil

8 drops of Angelica essential oil from the root

8 drops of essential oil of vetiver

3 Ounces Jojoba oil

Sweet Lady

Half Cup Sweet Almond Oil

12 drops of lavender essential oil

8 drops of sweet essential orange oil

4 drops of essential oil patchouli

Fresh leaves

Half Cup Sweet Almond Oil

8 drops of essential oil patchouli

8 drops of essential oil for cedar wood

8 drops of essential oil from spearmint

Fragrances for men and Colognes

The man in your life has to be smelling nice as well. Men love wearing colognes that they like , and also ones that the lady is in their lives too.

Try your hand to make your male friends some of these colognes. They'll not only smell great and feel great, but also you will feel secure knowing that they're all natural created scents.

Colognes can make people feel better and confident. Men tend to prefer woodsy and musky scents while others prefer gentler and more delicate scents.

Certain scents may be quite strong but they will make the men who is in your life smell amazing. Try experimenting with the recipes when one appears to be more overwhelming than the others.

Test these on the man in your life , and find out his opinion.

A man in the forest

5 drops of essential oil of the fir needle

3 drops of essential pine oil

5 drops of juniper berry essential oil

10 drops of essential oil from cedarwood

Pirate's treasure

10 drops of Bay West Indies essential oil

5 drops of sweet essential orange oil

5 drops of essential lime peel oil

3 drops of essential clove oil

Bros

10 drops of bergamot essential oil

3 drops of essential oil cardamom

5 drops of essential oil of patchouli

3 drops of essential oil for cedar wood

The Black Crow

10 drops of essential oil from black pepper

3 drops of essential clove oil

5 drops of essential oil sandalwood

3 drops of essential oil nutmeg

5 drops of essential lemon oil

Superman

5 drops in Atlas Cedar Wood essential oil

3 drops of essential oil from coriander

5 Drops of palmarosa essential oil

5 drops of essential ginger oil

5 drops of essential oil frankincense

The Lover

5 drops of essential oil from sandalwood

One Drop Vanilla Absolute

5 drops of essential lime peel oil

3 drops of essential oil of nutmeg

1 drop of essential oil of vetiver

5 drops of essential grapefruit oil

Nocturnal

10 drops of essential lavender oil

10 drops of essential oil for cedar wood

5 drops from sweet marjoram essential oils

One Drop Neroli essential oil

Orange Cologne

10 drops of essential lemon oil

10 drops of essential grapefruit oil

10 drops of essential basil oil

8 Ounces of Vodka

Man with a sense of sensual

10 drops of essential lavender oil

20 drops of essential oil from coriander

22 drops of essential oil from sandalwood

23 drops of essential oil for cedar wood

5 drops of essential oil of frankincense

100 ml vodka

Conclusion

Replace any products you have by making your own scents or body mists. Nature has given us incredible ingredients. You can utilize them all to create your own perfumes. If you have kids in the house These perfumes and body sprays could be dangerous. This book contains 35 recipe ideas that will be suitable for your family as well as you. It is possible to make your own perfume using these recipes, and enhance your health as well as the atmosphere of your home.

There are recipes that can be used to create solid scents since the essential oils are readily available on the market. The commercial perfumes might contain chemicals that can be damaging to the skin. It is not necessary to purchase extravagant products as you can make your own organic perfumes at your own home. These perfumes are made with organic ingredients, and you might make a significant savings in dollars.

It's not difficult to make a natural scent however, you must buy gloves, tools, essential equipment containers, and molds to create them. It is essential to choose an area with adequate ventilation to protect yourself from the smoke and evaporation of certain recipes. The book offers recipes for making various kinds of scents that help protect your skin from allergic reactions.

www.ingramcontent.com/pod-product-compliance
Lightning Source LLC
Chambersburg PA
CBHW050727030426
42336CB00012B/1443